Alkaline Cancer Diet

A Working Guide and 21-Day Meal Plan for Fighting Cancer and Healing Naturally

By

Elizabeth. A. Cohen

Alkaline Cancer Diet

Copyright © 2019

All rights reserved. This book or any portion thereof may not be reproduced or used in any manner whatsoever without the express written permission of the publisher except for the use of brief quotations in a book review.

ISBN: 9781697110210

Warning and Disclaimer

Every effort has been made to make this book as accurate as possible. However, no warranty or fitness is implied. The information provided is on an "as-is" basis. The author and the publisher shall have no liability or responsibility to any person or entity with respect to any loss or damages that arise from the information in this book.

MEDICAL DISCLAIMER: I am not a medical doctor and I do not advise that you stop cancer treatment to pursue an alkaline diet. The information available in this book is from my own personal research and it has not been endorsed by the medical field.

Publisher contact

Skinny Bottle Publishing

books@skinnybottle.com

- Introduction 5
- Chapter 1 7
- Common Cancer Symptoms 7
  - Lump in the breast or elsewhere on your body 8
  - Chest pain, coughing, and breathlessness 8
  - Change in bowel habits 8
  - Bleeding 8
  - Moles 9
  - Unexplained weight loss 9
- Chapter 2 10
- Cancer: Treatment and Prevention 10
  - Radiation 11
  - Chemotherapy 11
  - Surgery 11
  - Hormone Therapy 12
  - Gene Therapy 12
  - Immunotherapy 13
  - Preventing Cancer 13
- Chapter 3 15
- Alkaline and Cancer 15
- Chapter 4 19
- High Alkaline Cancer Fighting Foods 19
  - Onion 19

    Using Onions: You can add onions to any meal or consume it as a soup..................20

    Lemons 20

    Kale 21

    Turmeric 22

    Garlic 23

    Ginger 25

    Brussels Sprouts 26

    Avocado 27

    Seeds and nuts 29

    Mushrooms 30

    Oregano 30

Chapter 6 32

21 Day Cancer-Fighting Alkaline Diet 32

    Breakfast recipes 32

    Lunch Recipes 51

    Dinner Recipes 73

    Dessert recipes 98

    Drink Recipes 118

Conclusion 127

Introduction

There is a reason why you are reading this book, you are either suffering from cancer, you know someone who suffers from cancer or you have simply taken an interest in the subject. Regardless of the category that you fall under cancer is a devastating disease. Cancer kills approximately 7.6 million people worldwide per year. It continues to have a major impact across the globe. There are over 200 different types of cancer; however, the most common cancers are:

- Pancreatic cancer
- Endometrial cancer
- Leukemia
- Kidney cancer
- Renal pelvis cancer
- Thyroid cancer
- Non-Hodgkin lymphoma
- Melanoma of the skin
- Bladder cancer
- Rectum and colon cancer

- Bronchus cancer
- Breast cancer

Cancer is a condition where cells in certain parts of the body reproduce and grow uncontrollably. The cancerous cells destroy and invade surrounding organs and healthy tissue. Cancer will start in one part of the body and if it isn't diagnosed quickly, it will spread to other areas. This process is referred to as metastasis. More than one in three people will suffer from some form of cancer in their lifetime.

In the preceding chapters you will learn about the symptoms, treatment, and prevention of cancer as well as information on how to start an alkaline diet.

Chapter 1

Common Cancer Symptoms

It is important to pay attention to any sudden changes within your body, these include the following:

- Bowel habits
- Blood in urine
- The appearance of a lump

These symptoms may not be cancerous because they are linked to other illnesses; however, if you are experiencing any of them it is important that you visit your doctor to rule out cancer. If cancer is suspected, you will be referred to a specialist at the earliest possible date. You will then have further tests such as an X-ray or a biopsy. Here is a list of the most common cancer symptoms.

Lump in the breast or elsewhere on your body

If you notice a lump in your breast, go and see your doctor immediately. Your doctor will examine you; however, if they suspect cancer you will be referred to a specialist.

Chest pain, coughing, and breathlessness

If you have had a cough for more than three weeks, go and visit your doctor. Symptoms such as not being able to breathe properly or chest pains are also signs of pneumonia. Go and see your doctor immediately if you are experiencing any of these symptoms.

Change in bowel habits

If you are experiencing any of the following changes and they have lasted for more than a few weeks go and see your doctor.

- Blood in your stools
- Constipation or diarrhea for no reason
- Still feeling as if you need to use to the toilet after emptying your bowels
- Pain in the anus or stomach
- Continuous bloating

Bleeding

If you have any unexplained bleeding or blood, go and see your doctor.

- Blood in the urine
- Bleeding when you are not on your period
- Bleeding from the anus
- Coughing up blood
- Blood in your vomit

Moles

Go and visit your doctor if you have a mole that:

- Has an asymmetrical or irregular shape
- Has jagged or irregular border
- Has different colors, it might be white and pink or black and brown
- Is larger than 7mm in diameter
- Is bleeding, crusting or itchy

If you are experiencing any of the above there is a chance that you might have a type of skin cancer called malignant melanoma.

Unexplained weight loss

If you are losing weight without making an effort through diet and exercise or through stress you will need to see your doctor straight away.

Chapter 2

Cancer: Treatment and Prevention

Cancer treatment is dependent upon a number of factors such as the type of cancer, health status, age, how much cancer has spread and other personal characteristics. There is no standard cancer treatment, and patients will often receive a combination of palliative care and therapies. Treatment typically falls into one of the following categories:

- Radiation
- Chemotherapy
- Surgery
- Hormone therapy
- Gene therapy
- Immunotherapy

Radiation

Radiation treatment is also referred to as radiotherapy. It attacks cancer by targeting cancer cells with high-energy rays. This process damages the molecules and causes them to self destruct. Radiotherapy uses high-energy gamma rays which are sent through metals such as radium or high-energy x-rays. Radiation treatment during the early stage of cancer can cause serious side effects because it damages healthy normal tissue.

Chemotherapy

Chemotherapy involves using chemicals that corrupt the process of cell division which damages DNA or proteins. As with radiation therapy, chemotherapy causes cancer cells to self destruct. It is used to treat cancer that has spread throughout the body and is often used on lymphoma and leukemia. Chemotherapy treatment takes place in cycles giving the body time to heal. Common side effects include vomiting, fatigue, nausea, and hair loss.

Surgery

Surgery is the most common form of treatment for cancer that has not spread. It is possible to cure a patient by cutting cancer out of the body. This is typically seen in the removal of a testicle, breast or the prostate. Once the disease has spread, surgery may no longer be possible.

The surgical procedure continues to develop with new technologies such as iKnife which sniffs out cancer. At present, when a tumor is removed from the body, the surgeon will also remove healthy tissue to make sure that there have been no malignant cells left behind. This means that the patient is kept under anesthetic for a further 30 minutes while the tissue sample is tested to make sure that all cancer cells have been removed. After the test, if it is found that there are more cancer cells the surgeon will have to remove more tissue. According to the Imperial College of London science team, the iKnife could eliminate the need to send samples for testing.

A study conducted by the Washington University School of Medicine discovered that they could locate cancer cells using high-resolution glasses. The tumor is injected with a fluorescent marker that only attaches to cancerous cells. Under a special light, the cancer cells glow blue in color. This makes it easier for doctors to remove cancer cells.

Hormone Therapy

A number of cancers such as prostate and breast cancer have been linked to certain hormones. The aim of hormone therapy is to alter the production of the hormone in the body to stop the cancer cells from growing or to kill them completely. Hormone therapies for breast cancer focus on reducing levels of estrogen and prostate cancer hormone therapies focus on reducing levels of testosterone.

Gene Therapy

Gene therapy replaces genes that have been damaged with healthy genes that are used to discover the root cause of cancer. Other gene therapies are focused on damaging the DNA of the cancer cell so that it self destructs. Gene therapy is still in the testing phases.

Immunotherapy

Studies have found that it is possible to clone the patient's cells to improve their immune system so that cancer cells are destroyed naturally.

Preventing Cancer

There are some cancers that are linked to lifestyle choices; these include alcohol consumption and smoking tobacco. Choosing not to indulge in these behaviors will reduce the risk of liver, mouth, throat and lung cancer. People who currently use tobacco and alcohol can reduce their risks by quitting.

You can prevent skin cancer by staying out of the sun and protecting yourself by using sun cream, wearing a hat, and a shirt. Cancer is also linked to dietary habits and physicians recommend diets that are low in fat and rich in vegetables fresh fruits and whole grains.

There are also some vaccinations that have been linked to preventing cancer. For example, apillomavirus vaccination is linked to cervical cancer. The Hepatitis B vaccine vaccinates against Hepatitis B which can cause liver cancer.

It is also advised that people are routinely screened for cancer to detect tumors or irregularities early even if there are no symptoms. Common screening methods for different cancers include:

- Pap smears
- Testicular self-examination
- Mammograms
- Breast self-examination

You can also reduce your risk of cancer by being physically active, reducing blood sugar levels, managing blood pressure and controlling cholesterol.

Chapter 3

Alkaline and Cancer

Year after year the public is asked to donate money to finding a cure for cancer and as yet, medical and scientific research has been unable to do so. On the other hand, there have been many successful alternative treatments that fail to gain approval and recognition from the medical field. Science has proved that a lot of illnesses stem from the irregular functioning of the digestive system and the negative effects that it has on the immune system and cancer is one of them.

When it comes to nutrition, the digestive system acts as a filter, the purpose of this filter is to sift the micronutrients out of the foods that we eat. However, when the filter cannot do its job because of unnatural ingredients such as the preservatives and additives that are present in our foods it gets blocked. This is why nutrition is such an important factor when it comes to healing the body.

Before we begin, I would like to define alkaline. Our bodies are constantly working to maintain the correct acid and alkaline balance, both of which have an effect on cancerous and healthy cells. Acidity and alkalinity are measured on a pH scale that ranges from 0-14, for those of you who were paying attention in your chemistry class, a Ph level that is less than 7 is acidic and more than 7 is alkaline. A Ph level of 7 is said to be neutral. At its core, an alkaline diet is based on foods and drinks that balance out the alkaline Ph levels in the body.

When the nutrients from our food get to our kidneys they produce either more bicarbonate (alkaline) ions or ammonium (acidic) ions. For our cells to be considered healthy our blood should have a pH of more than 7 which makes it slightly alkaline. The problem is that diets in the majority of western countries are highly acidic. Research has found that when the body has to overwork to neutralize the acid overload it has a negative impact on our health. This can lead to problems such as chronic diseases, skin problems, arthritis, allergies, inflammation, and cancer.

In the 1930s an effective and simple cancer treatment was developed, this treatment has been labeled as dangerous, experimental and alternative by the scientific and medical community which is why it is primarily referenced in publications that are not linked to the mainstream press.

The cancer treatment is known as alkaline therapy or pH therapy. The principles are very simple; when you lower or raise the internal pH level of a cancer cell you can stop it from progressing. When acid levels are increased in the body of a cancer patient, it causes a lot of pain because of the stress that is placed on normal cells. Therefore, the most effective therapy is a high pH therapy; this eliminates latent acidosis by normalizing the intracellular pH of the body. At the same time it increases the cancer cells' pH level to above 7.5, it is at this level that the cancer cells revert back to normal.

This treatment typically begins with an alkaline diet; there is a general consensus amongst medical practitioners and natural healers that changing the diet of a cancer patient is very beneficial after a diagnosis. The alkaline diet is a plant-based diet, it doesn't include the following:

- Wheat
- Dairy
- Sugar
- High gluten grains

The alkaline diet does promote the consumption of the following:

- Vegetable juices
- Lemons
- Limes
- Apples
- Broccoli
- Onions
- Avocado
- Asparagus

- Leafy green vegetables
- Dates
- Almonds
- Coconut water

All of which change the intracellular pH of the body so that it is as close to the ideal blood pH of 7.3/7.41. Whether you suffer from cancer or not, this should be a pH level that everyone aims for. Not only does an alkaline-based diet based on fruits and vegetables strengthen the immune system it creates an environment that prevents cancer cells from thriving.

It is shocking that the digestive system has been eliminated from the equation when it comes to conventional cancer treatment. Unfortunately, our nutrition has also been compromised by foods that are genetically modified and treated with herbicides and pesticides. It is also commonly known that foods such as processed sugar speed up the growth of cancer.

If you are not sure how to go about starting your alkaline cancer diet, the final chapter contains a detailed 21-day diet plan to get you started.

Chapter 4

High Alkaline Cancer Fighting Foods

As you have read, your diet is your number one weapon against fighting cancer and healing your body. Research suggests that less than one-third of all cancers are due to genetics, every other cancer is caused by factors such as personal choices, environment, and diet. You will drastically reduce your chances of becoming a cancer patient if you eat a healthy diet, avoid toxins and stay active. Whether you are battling cancer or not, here are 24 foods that will protect you against it.

Onion

Onions are a part of the allium family and they are high in sulfur and amino acids. Onions also contain quercetin which helps to rid the body of excess estrogen by detoxifying the liver. Onions also contain allicin which destroys fungi, viruses, bacteria and prevents cancer from developing. They also contain carminative herbs which benefit the digestive system.

Using Onions: You can add onions to any meal or consume it as a soup.

Onion Facts
- Prevent asthma and allergies
- Quercetin prevents the build-up of plaque on the arterial walls
- Reduces LDL cholesterol
- Reduces joint stiffness and swelling
- Reduces the risk of cancer
- Prevents the growth of tumors
- Reduces the risk of lung cancer in smokers
- Prevents heart disease
- Improves prostate health
- Limits the damage caused by bladder infections

Lemons

Lemons are a low carb fruit that contain enzymes that enhance nutrient absorption and contribute to the healthy function of the lungs, liver, intestines, and stomach.

Using Lemons: You can detoxify and alkalize the body by squeezing the juice of one lemon into a glass of water and drinking it as soon as you wake up. You can also use it to add flavor to food.

Lemon Facts

- Boosts the immune system
- Purifies the blood
- Reduces fever
- Aids in the weight loss process
- Relieves respiratory infections
- Relieves toothache
- Decreases blemishes and wrinkles
- Flushes out toxins
- Balances Ph levels
- A natural energizer
- Oxygenates the body

Kale

Kale is a part of the cruciferous vegetable family. Cruciferous vegetables are high in glucosinolates making them different from other vegetables. Glucosinolates destroy carcinogens before they cause any damage to our

DNA and prevent cancer cells from developing. Over the last few years, it has become popular in juice and smoothie shops, as well as a healthy snack. Kale is packed with minerals and vitamins such as iron, potassium, and calcium. It is also high in sulforaphane which is a type of isothiocyanate also found in Brussels sprouts, cauliflower, and broccoli. These powerful compounds prevent the activation of cancer cells, boost the immune system and enhance the body's natural detoxification process. Research has found that sulforaphane prevents the growth of tumors associated with cancer of the stomach, spleen, breast, colon, and prostate.

Eating Kale: To get the best out of its antioxidants and trace minerals, eat kale with a healthy source of fat such as grass-fed cheese, coconut oil or grass-fed butter. You should avoid eating it raw because its fibers are hard to digest and can cause digestive problems.

You can also juice kale and add it to a smoothie, for a healthy snack you can make kale chips by seasoning them and then roasting them in coconut oil.

Facts About Kale

- Lowers cholesterol
- Detoxifies the body

Turmeric

Turmeric is also known as golden milk; it contains a flavonoid called curcumin which is a powerful antioxidant that helps to regulate an abnormal immune system, reduce inflammation, and protects the body against cancer and other types of infection. It is a well-known fact that pharmaceutical companies attempt to imitate the same physiological pathways that turmeric has on the body in drugs such as ibuprofen and aspirin.

Using Tumeric: Turmeric can be consumed as a broth or tea. You can also add it to dishes such as stews and soups or use it to marinate meat or chicken.

Facts About Tumeric

- Reduces cholesterol
- Heals wounds
- Weight management
- Boosts the immune system
- Prevents cancer
- Controls diabetes
- Prevents liver disease
- Relieves arthritis
- Improves digestion
- Prevents Alzheimer's disease

Garlic

Garlic is another vegetable that contains allicin which protects the body against invasive substances and limits the amount of damage caused to the vascular system by reducing inflammation. Allicin also lowers cholesterol.

Research has found that garlic stabilizes blood glucose levels, improves the detoxification pathways and protects against bacteria and cancer.

Using Garlic

You can add garlic to any meal as it boosts the antioxidant protection present in all foods. You can make garlic even more effective by adding it to other foods that contain sulfur. It also acts as a powerful colon and oral probiotic. Make sure that you break or crush garlic before consuming it to activate the allinase enzyme to releases the allicin compound.

Facts About Garlic

- Anti-inflammatory
- Protects against clotting disorders and yeast infections
- Antibacterial and antiviral
- Daily intake reduces the risk of most cancers
- A good source of manganese, vitamin B6 and Vitamin C
- Improves blood pressure
- Protects against oxidative stress
- Helps to reduce blood sugar
- Reduces cholesterol and blood triglycerides
- Contains cardioprotective properties

- Helps to regulate fat cells
- A good source of selenium
- Improves iron metabolism

Olive Oil

Plant phenols protect the body in several ways, they are high in antioxidants and contain anti-inflammatory and anti-carcinogenic compounds.

Using Olive Oil: The main cause of sunburn and non-melanoma skin cancer is UV radiation. Apply olive oil to the skin before and after going out in the sun. You can also use it daily as a skin moisturizer.

Ginger

Ginger contains volatile oils that provide anti-fungal, anti-parasitic, anti-viral and anti-bacterial properties. According to research ginger stimulates the digestive system, relieves pain and increases the amount of glutathione produced by the body. Ginger's active components are 6-shogaol and 6-gingerol, both of which protect against liver and gastrointestinal cancer.

Using Ginger

You can add ginger to slaws, salads, dressings, marinades, stews, and soups. For an antioxidant-rich tonic, you can make fermented ginger ale, or steep it to make a hot brewed tea.

Facts About Ginger

- Suppresses coughs
- Prevents flu and cold
- Treats migraine
- Settles an upset stomach
- Prevents certain cancers
- Reduces menstrual pain
- Reduces arthritis pain
- Treats morning sickness
- Promotes a healthy heart
- Controls diabetes

Brussels Sprouts

Brussels are another cruciferous vegetable. They don't have the best reputation because of their smell when cooked. However, they are loaded with the following vitamins and nutrients:

- Vitamin A
- Vitamin B-6
- Vitamin C
- Vitamin K
- Manganese
- Potassium
- Folate

Brussels sprouts assist in building collagen which reduces wrinkles, they enhance the body's ability to absorb calcium and support the immune system.

Using Brussels

You can eat Brussels sprouts as a vegetable side dish with your meal. Roast or sauté them smothered in grass-fed butter or coconut oil and drizzle balsamic vinegar over them. You can also shave them and add Brussels sprouts to salads and slaws or steam and then puree them and season with salt, pepper, and turmeric to make hummus.

Facts About Brussels Sprouts

- 80 grams of Brussels sprouts contain more vitamin C than an orange
- Lower cholesterol
- Prevent colon cancer
- They contain sinigrin, a compound that fights against cancer
- A good source of protein
- Improve bone health
- Decrease the risk of obesity
- Decrease the risk of diabetes
- Decrease the risk of heart disease

Avocado

The most popular type of avocado is Haas; they are high in vital nutrients and phytochemicals such as:

- Dietary fiber
- Carotenoids
- Phytosterols
- Niacin
- Vitamins B-6, K, C, E
- Sodium
- Magnesium
- Potassium

Research has discovered that avocados benefit cardiovascular health by lowering total cholesterol in diabetes; they also improve blood lipid levels.

Using Avocados

Avocado can be used in a number of ways. You can add them to smoothies, use them to make guacamole, put them in an omelet or add them to a salad.

Facts about avocados

- One avocado contains twice as much potassium as a banana
- Reduce the risk of heart disease
- Enable the body to better absorb fat-soluble nutrients such as lutein and beta carotene.

Seeds and nuts

Seeds and nuts are a great source of phytosterols, manganese, biotin, fiber, magnesium and vitamin E, all of which are referred to as healthy fats. The American Heart Association refers to nuts as "little powerhouses of nutrition and taste"

Brazil nuts are one of the highest sources of selenium; sunflower seeds are also high in selenium which is a powerful immune-boosting mineral. Cashews contain the highest concentration of vitamin B and hazelnuts contain the highest concentration of folate, this is especially beneficial for women who are pregnant. Pistachios contain the highest concentration of phytosterols and almonds are known to lower total cholesterol. For extra omega 3 fatty acids add a mixture of flaxseeds, chia seeds and pumpkin seeds to your diet.

Using nuts

You can add nuts to desserts and salads or you can eat them as a healthy snack.

Facts about nuts

- Rich in flavonoids
- High in monosaturated fats
- Reduces bad cholesterol
- Maintains and raises good cholesterol
- High in vitamin E

- Helps with weight loss
- High in alpha-linolenic acid

Mushrooms

Mushrooms help with the absorption of calcium and other essential nutrients such as zinc, copper, riboflavin, choline, manganese, thiamine, and vitamin D because they contain bone fortifying nutrients.

Using Mushrooms

Prepare mushrooms in stuffed peppers, a hearty soup or toast them in olive oil and season with salt and pepper for a tasty side dish. You can trade your beef patty for a Portobello mushroom topped with avocado for a creamy topping. Make sure you don't overcook your mushrooms or you will lose most of the nutrients.

Oregano

Oregano is one of the many herbs that are high in antioxidants, consuming them on a daily basis is one of the easiest and most cost-effective things you can do to benefit your health. Herbs such as oregano are packed with nutrients as well as powerful anti-inflammatory components. It is a member of the Labiatae family and contains volatile oils that help to naturally detox the liver which eliminates compounds such as excess estrogen from the body. Oregano helps to prevent the development of cancer cells that cause ovarian, uterine, breast and prostate cancer.

Using Oregano

If you want to kill bacteria and boost the immune system oil of oregano is one of the most effective ways of doing so. You can take them as a supplement; you can also use oregano as a herb when cooking stews, soups, and salads.

Facts about oregano

- Protects against flu and cold viruses
- Helps to clear the airways and lungs of excess mucus
- Helps to stimulate the appetite.

Now that you have an informative list of powerful alkaline containing foods, it's time to move on to your diet plan.

Chapter 6

21 Day Cancer-Fighting Alkaline Diet

In this chapter, you will find breakfast, lunch, dinner, desserts and drinks list containing recipes that you can eat daily. Please note: I was only able to include 13 drink recipes due to space restrictions.

Breakfast recipes

1: Tasty Pumpkin Breakfast Bars

(Preparation time: 30 minutes/Serves: 4 servings)

Ingredients
- 2 cups of oats, gluten-free
- 1 cup of fresh pumpkin
- 1 teaspoon of vanilla

- 3 finely sliced pitted dates
- 1 teaspoon of cinnamon
- 2 tablespoons of chia seeds
- 1 tablespoon of hemp seeds
- ¼ cup of chopped raw almonds
- ¼ cup of shredded coconut flakes, unsweetened
- 1 teaspoon of coconut oil

Directions

1. Preheat the oven to 200 degrees C.
2. Grease a baking dish with coconut oil.
3. Combine the ingredients in a large mixing bowl.
4. Transfer the mixture into the pan and press it down.
5. Bake for 20 minutes until it becomes firm and golden brown in color.
6. Remove the tray from the oven and allow it to cool down for 1 hour.
7. Slice into bars and serve. Store the remainder in an airtight container for up to 3 days.

2: Muesli

(Preparation time: 8 hours /Serves: 2 servings)

Ingredients

- ½ a cup of rolled oats, gluten-free
- 1 cup of almond milk, unsweetened

- 1 tablespoon of sliced almonds
- ½ a cup of chopped apple
- A dash of cinnamon

Directions

1. Pour all the ingredients into a bowl and allow them to soak overnight in the fridge.

2. Add milk, and eat in the morning.

3: Berry Parfait

(Preparation time: 1 hour 10 minutes /Serves: 2 servings)

Ingredients

- ½ a cup of soaked cashews (soak for 1 hour)
- ½ a cup of unsweetened almond milk
- ½ a teaspoon of alcohol-free vanilla extract
- 1/3 cup of rolled oats, gluten-free
- 1 tablespoon of hemp seeds

Directions

1. Transfer the vanilla, coconut milk and cashews into a food processor and blend until smooth.

2. Transfer the ingredients into a small cup starting with the cashew cream, then the berries, top with the hemp seeds and oats and serve.

4: Berry Summer Smoothie

(Preparation time: 10 minutes/Serves: 1 serving)

Ingredients

- 1 large handful of spinach
- ½ a cup of mixed berries
- 1 frozen banana
- 1 freshly squeezed lime
- 1 teaspoon of cinnamon
- 1 tablespoon of coconut oil
- 1 tablespoon of chia seeds
- 1 cup of coconut water

Directions

1. Transfer all of the ingredients into a food processor and blend until smooth.
2. Pour into a glass and drink.

5: Fat Burning Smoothie

(Preparation time: 10 minutes/Serves: 1 serving)

Ingredients

- 1 cup of unsweetened almond milk
- 1 avocado
- 1 frozen banana
- 1 tablespoon of raw almond butter
- 1 teaspoon of chia seeds

- 1 handful of ice

Directions

1. Transfer all the ingredients into a food processor and blend until smooth.
2. Pour into a glass and serve.

6: Spiced Quinoa Breakfast

(Preparation time: 20 minutes/ Serves: 2 servings)

Ingredients

- 2 cups of unsweetened almond milk
- 1 cup of uncooked quinoa
- ½ a cup of chopped raw quinoa
- 2 tablespoons of hemp seeds
- 2 tablespoons of sunflower seeds (soaked overnight)
- 2 tablespoons of chia seeds
- 2 tablespoons of coconut flakes, unsweetened
- ½ a teaspoon of vanilla
- ¼ teaspoon of cinnamon
- A pinch of ground cloves
- A pinch of ground nutmeg
- A pinch of ground ginger
- 2 pitted dates

Directions

1. Transfer the dates and the almond milk into a food processor and blend to combine.

2. In a large saucepan add the quinoa, ginger, nutmeg, cloves, vanilla, cinnamon, and the date mixture. Stir to combine and heat for simmer at a low temperature for 10 minutes. Once cooked, take the saucepan off the cooker and let it sit for 5 minutes.

3. Divide the quinoa into bowls and top with chia seeds, blueberries, sunflower seeds, coconut flakes, hemp seeds, and almonds and serve.

7: Crunchy Almond Butter Smoothie

(Preparation time: 10 minutes/Serves: 2 servings)

Ingredients

- 2 cups of fresh spinach
- 2 cups of unsweetened almond milk
- 1 cup of frozen mixed berries
- 1 frozen banana
- 4 tablespoons of raw almond butter
- 1 tablespoon of chia seeds

Directions

1. Transfer all of the ingredients into a food processor and blend until smooth.

2. Pour into glasses and serve.

8: Lime Raspberry Smoothie

Preparation time: 10 minutes /Serves: 1 serving)

Ingredients

- 1 handful of spinach
- 1 cup of frozen raspberries
- 2 tablespoons of fresh lime juice
- 1 cup of unsweetened coconut milk
- 1 tablespoon of chia seeds

Directions

1. Transfer all of the ingredients into a food processor and blend until smooth.
2. Pour into a glass and serve.

9: Cinnamon Bun Smoothie

(Preparation time:10 minutes /Serves: 2 servings)

Ingredients

- 1 cup of coconut milk
- 1 handful of spinach (large)
- 1 frozen banana
- 2 tablespoons of raw almond butter
- 1 pitted date
- ¾ teaspoons of cinnamon
- 1 tablespoon of hemp seeds

- 1 scoop of coconut vanilla flavor Organic Alkamind Daily Protein
- 1 cup of ice cubes

Directions

1. Transfer all the ingredients into a food processor and blend until smooth.
2. Pour into glasses and serve.

10: Cacao Protein Smoothie

(Preparation time: 10 minutes/Serves: 1 serving)

Ingredients

- 1 cup of spinach
- ½ a cup of raw almonds, soaked overnight
- ¼ cup of ground flaxseed
- ¼ cup of raw cacao powder
- 1 frozen banana
- ½ a cup of frozen blueberries
- 1 teaspoon of freshly squeezed lemon juice
- ¼ teaspoon of Celtic Grey sea salt
- 1 cup of almond milk
- 1 scoop of Organic Alkamind Daily Protein, creamy chocolate flavor

Directions

1. Transfer all ingredients into a food processor and blend until smooth.

2. Pour into a glass and drink.

11: Seeded Super Pancakes

(Preparation time: 15 minutes/Serves: 3 servings)

Ingredients

- ¼ cup of pumpkin seeds
- ¼ cup of sesame seeds
- ¼ cup of flax seeds
- ½ a cup of chia seeds
- 1 cup of buckwheat oats
- 1 ½ teaspoon of ground cinnamon
- ½ a teaspoon of baking powder
- 1 teaspoon of baking soda
- ¼ teaspoon of fine Celtic Grey sea salt
- ½ a teaspoon of stevia extract
- 2 tablespoons of almond milk
- 1 teaspoon of coconut oil
- Lemon juice
- Stevia

Directions

1. Combine the first five ingredients in a food processor and blend them into a flour

2. Pour 2 cups of the flour into a large bowl.

3. Add the rest of the ingredients except the coconut oil and whisk to combine.

4. Heat the coconut oil in a non-stick frying pan over high heat.

5. Pour a thin layer of the batter into the frying pan and cook for 2 minutes on both sides.

6. Repeat until all the batter has been used.

7. Transfer onto plates and serve with lemon juice and stevia.

12: Quinoa Porridge

(Preparation time: 15 minutes/Serves: 1 serving)

Ingredients

- ½ a cup of quinoa flakes
- 1 tablespoon of chia seeds
- 1 tablespoon of coconut oil
- ¼ cup of almond milk
- ¼ teaspoon of ground cinnamon
- ¼ teaspoon of stevia extract
- 1 handful of crushed walnuts

Directions

1. Soak the chia seeds in 3 tablespoons of water for 10 minutes.

2. Add the quinoa flakes ¼ cups of water, stir to combine and microwave for 2 ½ minutes.

3. Add the stevia, cinnamon, almond milk, coconut oil, and chia seeds and stir to combine.

4. Top with crushed walnuts and eat.

13: Blueberry Porridge

(Preparation time: 15 minutes/Serves: 1 serving)

Ingredients

- ¼ cup of buckwheat oats soaked overnight.
- 1 tablespoon of chia seeds soaked overnight
- 10 almonds soaked overnight
- ½ a cup of unsweetened almond milk
- ¼ teaspoon of ground cinnamon
- ¼ teaspoon of vanilla extract
- Stevia
- Blueberries

Directions

1. Rinse the buckwheat and combine it with the almond milk in a saucepan. Cook for 7 minutes, it should become creamy and cracked.

2. Add the stevia, vanilla extract, cinnamon, chia seeds, and almonds and stir to combine.

3. Pour into a bowl, top with blueberries and eat.

14: Chocolate Chia Pudding

(Preparation time: 12 hours 15 minutes/Serves: 1 serving)

Ingredients

- ¼ cup of chia seeds
- 1 teaspoon of vanilla extract
- 1 tablespoon of cacao powder
- 1/8 teaspoon of Celtic Grey sea salt
- 1/8 teaspoon of ground cinnamon
- ¼ teaspoon of stevia extract
- 1 ¼ cup of unsweetened almond milk

Directions

1. Transfer all of the ingredients into a mixing bowl and stir to combine.
2. Pour the ingredients into a mason jar, seal the lid and leave in the fridge overnight.
3. The next morning, stir and eat for breakfast.

15: Fennel Mint Smoothie

(Preparation time: 10 minutes/Serves: 1 serving)

Ingredients

- 1 chopped cucumber
- 2 cups of spinach
- ½ a chopped fennel bulb

- ¼ cup of fresh mint leaves
- 1 chopped avocado
- 1 tablespoon of chia seeds
- 30 grams of pea protein and sprouted rice powder
- ½ a cup of coconut water
- ½ a cup of ice

Directions

1. Transfer all ingredients into a food processor and blend until smooth.
2. Pour into a glass and drink.

16: Super Alkaline Shake

(Preparation time: 10 minutes/Serves: 1 serving)

Ingredients

- 1 cucumber
- 2 large kale leaves, remove the stalks
- ½ an ounce of fresh ginger
- 1 avocado
- ½ a cup of coconut water
- ¼ cup of fresh mint
- 1 tablespoon of fresh parsley
- The juice of 1 lime
- 1 teaspoon of coconut oil

- 1 tablespoon of chia seeds soaked overnight
- ¼ teaspoon of stevia

Directions

1. Transfer all ingredients into a food processor and blend until smooth.
2. Pour into a glass and drink.

17: Breakfast: Granola

(Preparation time: 1 hour 30 minutes /Serves: 2 servings)

Ingredients

- 2 cups of raw almonds
- 2 cups of raw cashews
- 2 cups of raw almonds
- 1 cup of shredded coconut flakes unsweetened
- ¼ cup of dried organic blueberries
- ¼ cup of organic golden berries

Ingredients for the granola syrup

- 3 tablespoons of cold-pressed coconut oil
- 1/3 cup of coconut liquid nectar
- 2 tablespoons of filtered water
- ½ a teaspoon of cinnamon powder
- ½ a teaspoon of Celtic Grey sea salt
- 1 teaspoon of vanilla extract

Directions

1. Preheat the oven to 300 degrees C.

2. Transfer the nuts into a food processor and blend to chop them into small pieces.

3. Transfer the nuts into a large bowl and add the dried berries and coconut flakes.

4. Combine the ingredients for the granola syrup in a small mixing bowl and whisk to combine.

5. Pour the syrup onto the nuts and stir to combine.

6. Arrange the granola onto a baking tray and bake for 20 minutes. After 10 minutes remove the tray from the oven and stir and then continue to bake.

7. Once cooked, remove the granola from the oven and allow it to cool for 1 hour and then transfer it to an airtight container for storage.

8. Serve with raw almond or coconut milk.

18: Avocado Detox Smoothie

(Preparation time: 10 minutes/Serves: 1 serving)

Ingredients

- 1 cup of coconut water
- 1 Hass avocado, peeled, deseeded and sliced
- 1 cucumber, sliced
- 1 bunch of fresh spinach, chopped
- 1 piece of ginger (1-inch thick), chopped

Directions

1. Put all the ingredients into a food processor and blend until smooth.
2. Pour into a glass and serve.

19: Breakfast: Pumpkin Pie Bowl

(Preparation time: /Serves: 2 servings)

Ingredients

- ½ a cup of cashews
- ¾ cup of canned organic pumpkin puree
- 1 tablespoon of coconut oil
- ¼ cup of filtered water
- ¼ teaspoon of Celtic Grey sea salt
- ¼ teaspoon of finely diced star anise spice
- ¼ teaspoon of cinnamon
- 2 small dates
- ½ a teaspoon of vanilla
- ½ a teaspoon of fresh chopped ginger

Ingredients for the granola crumble

- ½ a cup of raw almonds
- ½ a cup of almond flakes unsweetened
- ½ a cup of pitted dates

Directions for the granola crumble

1. Transfer all of the ingredients into a food processor and blend for 60 seconds.

2. Pour the mixture into a bowl and set it to one side.

Directions for the filler

1. Transfer all of the ingredients into a food processor and blend until smooth.

2. Pour the filler on top of the granola and then put the bowl in the fridge for an hour to thicken.

3. When ready to serve garnish with nutmeg or cinnamon and crushed almonds and hemp seeds.

20: Breakfast: Spicy Pumpkin Smoothie

(Preparation time: 10 minutes/Serves: 2 servings)

Ingredients

- 2 cups of unsweetened almond milk
- 1 cup of baby spinach
- 1 cup of organic unsweetened pumpkin
- 1 frozen banana
- 1 teaspoon of cinnamon
- ¼ teaspoon of minced ginger root powder
- ¼ teaspoon of nutmeg
- 1 date
- 1 tablespoon of chia seeds

Directions

1. Blend the almond milk and the spinach in a food processor.

2. Add the rest of the ingredients except the chia seeds and continue to blend until smooth.

3. Add the chia seeds and blend on low. Let it sit for 10 minutes.

4. Pour into glasses and serve.

21: Coconut Banana Smoothie

(Preparation time: 10 minutes/Serves: 1 serving)

Ingredients

- 2 cups of fresh spinach
- 2 cups of unsweetened coconut milk
- 1 green apple
- 1 frozen banana
- 1/3 cup of rolled oats, gluten-free
- 1 scoop of Daily Protein, Vanilla Coconut
- 1 tablespoon of coconut oil
- 1 tablespoon of flax seeds
- ½ a teaspoon of cinnamon

Directions

1. Pour all ingredients into a food processor and blend until smooth.

2. Pour out into a glass and serve.

Lunch Recipes

1: Basil Mint Avocado Gazpacho

(Preparation time:15 minutes /Serves: 2 servings)

Ingredients

- ½ a cup of extra virgin olive oil
- 2 handfuls of fresh basil
- 1 handful of fresh mint
- 1 ripe avocado, Haas
- 1 cucumber, remove the seeds
- 2 cloves of garlic
- 3 green onions, remove the roots
- 2 cups of filtered water
- The juice of 1 lime
- 2 teaspoons of Celtic Grey sea salt

Directions

1. For the garnish, take ¼ of the basil and mint leaves, add them to a food processor, add the olive oil and blend to combine. Transfer into a small bowl and set it to one side.

2. Put the rest of the ingredients into the food processor and blend until smooth.

3. Transfer into bowls, garnish with the mint and basil and serve.

2: Avocado Creamy Hummus

(Preparation time: 15 minutes /Serves: 2 servings)

Ingredients

- 2 organic avocados, Haas
- 1 can of white beans
- The juice from 1 lime
- 1 tablespoon of extra virgin olive oil
- ½ a teaspoon of Celtic Grey sea salt
- ¼ teaspoon of cayenne pepper
- Cucumber, celery, carrot or bell pepper cut into sticks

Directions

1. Transfer all of the ingredients into a food processor and blend until smooth.

2. Serve with cucumber, carrots, celery or bell pepper sticks.

3: Sharp and Sweet Summer Salad

(Preparation time:20 minutes/ Serves: 4 servings)

Ingredients for the salad

- Butter lettuce, 1 large head, chopped
- Green beans, 1 handful, sliced into ¼ inch coins
- 1 shredded beet
- 1 chopped peach

- ¼ cup of shelled pistachios

Ingredients for the dressing

- ¼ cup of lemon juice, freshly squeezed
- ½ a cup of extra virgin olive oil
- 1 clove of minced garlic
- 1 small handful of chopped basil

Directions

1. Combine the ingredients for the dressing in a small bowl and whisk them together thoroughly.
2. Transfer all the ingredients for the salad into a large salad bowl and toss to combine.
3. Coat with the salad dressing and toss to combine.
4. Divide onto dishes and serve.

4: Beetroot Cabbage and Apple Salad

(Preparation time: 20 minutes/Serves: 2 servings)

Ingredients for the salad

- 1 chopped butter lettuce head
- 1 spiralized green apple
- 1 spiralized small beet
- 1 cup of purple cabbage, chopped
- 2 tablespoons of hemp seeds
- 2 tablespoons of sunflower seeds

Ingredients for the dressing

- 1/4 cup of freshly squeezed lemon juice
- 2 tablespoons of apple cider vinegar
- 2/3 cup of extra virgin olive oil
- ¼ cup of chopped cilantro
- 1 teaspoon of black pepper
- Celtic Grey sea salt

Directions

1. Transfer the ingredients for the dressing into a small bowl, season with salt and whisk together thoroughly.

2. Transfer the salad into a large bowl and toss to combine.

3. Divide onto plates, drizzle the salad dressing over the top and serve.

5: *Avocado Wraps*

(Preparation time: 20 minutes /Serves: 4 servings)

Ingredients

- 4 lettuce leaves
- 2 sliced avocados
- 1 large handful of chopped spinach
- 2 diced tomatoes
- 4 teaspoons of chopped cilantro

- 1 diced red onion
- 1 teaspoon of cumin
- Celtic Grey sea salt
- Green jalapeno pepper (optional)
- Alfafa sprouts (optional)

Directions

1. Spread the avocado on the lettuce leaves, arrange the rest of the ingredients on top.
2. Fold in half and serve.

6: Ginger Carrot and Avocado Salad

(Preparation time: 20 minutes /Serves: 4 servings)

Ingredients for the salad

- 1 head of chopped romaine lettuce
- 1 sliced Haas avocado
- 1 diced red bell pepper
- ½ a chopped red onion
- 1 diced tomato

Ingredients for the dressing

- ¼ cup of filtered water
- 2 tablespoons of freshly squeezed lemon
- 1 tablespoon of extra virgin olive oil
- 1 teaspoon of tahini

- ½ a teaspoon of toasted sesame oil
- 1 tablespoon of wheat-free tamari
- ½ a cup of chopped carrots
- 2 tablespoons of chopped ginger
- ¼ teaspoon of Celtic Grey sea salt
- 1 date
- 1 teaspoon of apple cider vinegar

Directions

1. Transfer all of the ingredients for the dressing into a food processor and blend until smooth.

2. Combine all the ingredients for the salad into a large salad bowl, pour the dressing over the top and toss to combine.

3. Divide onto plates and serve.

7: Cucumber, Watermelon, and Avocado Salad

(Preparation time:20 minutes /Serves: 2 servings)

Ingredients

- 2 sliced avocados
- 1 small cubed watermelon
- 2 cucumbers peeled and chopped into 1-inch pieces
- 1 diced tomato
- 1 tablespoon of extra virgin olive oil
- 2 tablespoons of freshly squeezed lime juice

- 1/3 cup of chopped cilantro
- Celtic Grey sea salt
- Black pepper
- 1 handful of arugula (optional)

Directions

1. Combine the avocado, lime juice and olive oil in a medium-sized bowl and toss to combine.

2. In a large bowl, combine the cilantro, cucumber, and watermelon and toss to combine.

3. Add the avocado mixture and season with salt and pepper.

4. Divide onto plates and serves.

8: Mint Green Basil Salad

(Preparation time:20 minutes /Serves: 4 servings)

Ingredients

- 1 chopped head of romaine lettuce
- 1 yellow or red sliced bell pepper
- ½ a chopped red onion
- 1 diced tomato

Ingredients for the dressing

- ¼ cup of filtered water
- 2 teaspoons of freshly squeezed lemon juice
- 3 teaspoons of tahini

- 1 teaspoon of coconut liquid nectar
- 1 tablespoon of chopped onion
- ¼ cup of loosely packed parsley
- 1/8 cup of basil
- 1/8 cup of mint
- 1 clove of garlic
- 1 tablespoon of extra virgin olive oil
- ½ a teaspoon of Celtic Grey sea salt

Directions

1. Transfer the ingredients for the dressing into a food processor and blend until smooth.

2. Combine the ingredients for the salad into a large salad bowl, pour the dressing over the top and toss to combine.

3. Divide onto plates and serve.

9: Avocado French Fries

(Preparation time: 30 minutes /Serves: 1 serving)

Ingredients

- 2 Haas organic avocados
- ¼ cup of sesame seeds
- 2 teaspoons of Celtic Grey sea salt

Directions

1. Preheat the oven to 200 degrees C.

2. Slice the avocados into the shape of French fries.

3. Blend the salt and the sesame seeds in a NutriBullet until it turns into a powder. Pour the powder onto a plate.

4. Dip the avocados strips into the powder so they are completely covered.

5. Line a baking tray with parchment paper.

6. Arrange the coated avocados on the baking tray and bake for 20 minutes.

7. Remove from the oven and eat.

10: Green Detox Soup

(Preparation time: 10 minutes /Serves: 4 servings)

Ingredients

- 2 cups of filtered water
- 2 chopped medium cucumbers
- ½ a bunch of chopped spinach
- 2 chopped celery stalks
- ¼ cup of freshly squeezed lemon juice
- ¼ cup of extra virgin olive oil
- 1 clove of garlic
- 1 teaspoon of Celtic Grey sea salt

Directions

1. Transfer all ingredients into a food processor and blend until smooth.

2. Pour into bowls, garnish with basil and serve.

11: Lunch: Butternut Squash Creamy Soup

(Preparation time: 30 minutes/Serves: 2 servings)

Ingredients

- ¼ cup of filtered water
- 1 finely chopped onion
- 2 pounds of chopped and peeled butternut squash
- 1 chopped carrot
- 1 ½ inch of grated fresh ginger
- ½ a teaspoon of cinnamon
- 1 cup of almond milk
- 1 tablespoon of ground coriander
- 3 cups of yeast-free vegetable broth
- Celtic Grey sea salt
- Black pepper

Directions

1. Sauté the onions in a large pan over medium heat for 5 minutes until they turn golden brown in color.

2. Add the coriander, cinnamon, ginger, carrot, and squash.

3. Cook for a further 8 minutes stirring occasionally.

4. Add the almond milk and the vegetable broth and bring the ingredients to a boil for 30 minutes stirring occasionally.

5. Pour the ingredients into a food processor and blend until it becomes smooth.

6. Add some salt and pepper, divide into bowls and serve.

12: Lunch: Quinoa Salad

(Preparation time: 30 minutes/ Serves: 4 servings)

Ingredients

- 1 cup of quinoa
- 2 cups of filtered water
- 1 can of adzuki beans
- 1 finely diced red bell pepper
- 1 diced avocado
- 1 bunch of sliced scallions
- 6 tablespoons of extra virgin olive oil
- 2 tablespoons of lime juice
- 2 tablespoons of chopped cilantro
- 1 teaspoon of cumin
- Celtic Grey sea salt
- Black pepper
- Chopped red onion for garnish (optional)

Directions

1. Combine the water, quinoa and a pinch of salt in a medium saucepan. Cover and simmer over low heat until the water has been absorbed. This should take approximately 15 minutes. Take the saucepan off the cooker and set it to one side.

2. To make the dressing combine the olive oil, cumin, lime juice and a pinch of salt in a small bowl and whisk to combine.

3. In a large bowl combine the cilantro, avocado, red bell pepper, adzuki beans, scallions, and the quinoa. Stir to combine.

4. Pour the dressing over the quinoa, stir to combine and serve.

13: Lunch: Avocado and Sweet Potato Soup

(Preparation time: 1 hour /Serves: 2 servings)

Ingredients

- 1 cup of cooked mashed sweet potato
- ½ a cup of yeast-free vegetable broth
- ½ a cup of almond milk
- ½ a can of white beans
- ½ a teaspoon of chipotle powder
- ½ a teaspoon of cumin
- ¼ teaspoon of Celtic Grey sea salt
- 1/8 teaspoon of chili powder

- ½ a Hass avocado, diced
- The juice of 1 wedge of lime
- ½ a cup of chopped parsley
- 1 teaspoon of thyme leaves
- ½ a teaspoon of diced jalapeno (optional)

Directions

1. Preheat the oven to 400 degrees F.
2. Wash the sweet potato and then bake until tender. This should take approximately 45 minutes.
3. Once cooked, removed the sweet potatoes from the oven, remove the skin and place them into a food processor. Add the almond milk, beans, and vegetable broth. Blend until smooth.
4. Add the spices and the salt and continue to blend.
5. Pour into bowls and garnish with thyme leaves, parsley, spinach, avocado, and lime juice.

13: Green Goddess With Cumin and Avocado Dressing

(Preparation time: 30 minutes/Serves: 2 servings)

Ingredients

- 3 cups of chopped kale
- ½ a cup of chopped broccoli florets
- 1 cup of zucchini
- 1/3 cup of halved cherry tomatoes, halved

- 2 tablespoons of hemp seeds

Ingredients for the cumin avocado dressing

- 1 Hass avocado
- 1 tablespoon of cumin powder
- The juice of 2 limes
- 1 cup of filtered water
- ¼ teaspoon of Celtic Grey sea salt
- 1 tablespoon of extra virgin olive oil
- A dash of cayenne pepper
- ¼ teaspoon of smoked paprika (optional)

Ingredients for the Tahini Lemon Dressing

- ¼ cup of tahini
- ½ a cup of filtered water
- The juice of ½ a lemon
- 1 clove of minced garlic
- ¾ teaspoon of Celtic Grey sea salt
- 1 tablespoon of extra virgin olive oil
- Black pepper

Directions

1. Steam the kale and the broccoli for 4 minutes.

2. Use a spiralizer to create the zucchini noodles, place them into a large bowl, add the cherry tomatoes and the cumin avocado dressing, toss to combine.

3. Arrange the steamed broccoli and kale onto plates and drizzle the lemon tahini dressing over the top.

4. Top with the zucchini noodles and tomatoes, sprinkle with hemp seeds and serve.

14: Pomegranate and Spinach Salad With Lemon Tarragon Dressing

(Preparation time: 30 minutes /Serves: 2 servings)

Ingredients

- 4 cups of baby spinach
- 1/3 cup of pomegranate seeds
- 2 thinly sliced baby leeks
- 1 diced Haas avocado
- ½ a cup of rinsed and drained white beans
- ¼ cup of pine nuts

Ingredients for the dressing

- 2 tablespoons of freshly squeezed lemon juice
- 1 tablespoon of freshly grated lemon zest
- ½ a cup of extra virgin olive oil
- 2 cloves of minced garlic
- 2 tablespoons of fresh chopped tarragon
- ½ a teaspoon of Celtic Grey sea salt
- Black pepper

Directions

1. Combine all the salad ingredients into a large bowl.

2. Combine all the dressing ingredients in a small bowl and whisk to combine.

3. Pour the dressing over the salad and toss to combine.

4. Arrange onto plates and serve.

15: Fresh Greens and Creamy Herb Dressing

(Preparation time:30 minutes/ Serves: 2 servings)

Ingredients

- 1 cup of filtered water
- 1 cup of raw cashews
- ¼ cup of extra virgin olive oil
- 2 tablespoons of freshly squeezed lemon juice
- 1 teaspoon of Celtic Grey sea salt
- 1 large pitted date
- 1 tablespoon of roughly chopped oregano
- 1 tablespoon of roughly chopped basil
- 1 tablespoon of roughly chopped sage
- 1 tablespoon of roughly chopped dill

Ingredients for the salad

- 1 bunch of Romaine lettuce or spinach
- 1 diced Hass avocado
- ½ a sliced red onion

Directions

1. Transfer all the ingredients for the dressing except for the herbs into a food processor and blend until smooth.

2. Add the herbs and continue to blend.

3. Season with salt and pepper and blend again.

4. Add the salad ingredients into a large bowl and toss to combine.

5. Divide the salad onto plates, drizzle with the dressing and serve.

16: Collard Green Rolls

(Preparation time: 30 minutes/Serves: 4 servings)

Ingredients for the filling

- 1 large collard green with the thick part of the stem cut off
- ½ a cucumber sliced into matchsticks
- 1 carrot sliced into matchsticks
- ½ a sliced Haas avocado
- 1 small handful of mung bean sprouts
- 2 sprigs of chopped basil
- 4 sprigs of chopped mint
- 1 small handful of chopped cilantro

Ingredients for the dipping sauce

- 1 teaspoon of minced ginger
- 1 clove of minced garlic
- 1 sliced green onion
- ¼ cup of Tamari, gluten-free

Directions

1. Combine the ingredients for the dipping sauce into a small bowl. Whisk together thoroughly and set to one side.

2. Arrange the collard greens out on a chopping board, place the filling in the middle, roll it up like a burrito and serve with the dipping sauce.

17: Creamy Broccoli Soup

(Preparation time: 30 minutes/Serves: 4 servings)

Ingredients

- 4 cups of yeast-free vegetable broth
- 1 large head of broccoli cut into florets
- 1 can of garbanzo beans, drained and rinsed
- 3 cloves of minced garlic
- 1 chopped onion
- 1 peeled sweet potato sliced into chunks
- 1 teaspoon of dried thyme
- 1 teaspoon of whole celery seeds
- 1 ½ teaspoon of salt

- ½ a teaspoon of dried marjoram
- ¼ teaspoon of ground black pepper
- ¼ teaspoon of turmeric powder

Directions

1. In a large saucepan combine the garbanzo beans, black pepper, turmeric, marjoram, thyme, celery seeds, garlic, onion, sweet potato, and vegetable broth. Cook the ingredients over medium heat, put a lid on the saucepan and simmer for 20 minutes. Once the vegetables have become tender, take the saucepan off the stove.

2. Pour the ingredients into a food processor in batches and blend until smooth.

3. Pour the soup back into the saucepan, season with salt, stir, cover and allow it to simmer for 10 minutes.

4. Divide into bowls and serve.

18: Sweet Potato Curried Soup

(Preparation time: 30/Serves:4 servings)

Ingredients

- 1 tablespoon of coconut oil
- 1 piece of crushed ginger, 1 ½ inch
- 4 cloves of minced garlic
- The juice and zest of 1 lime
- 2 teaspoons of curry

- 3 sweet potatoes, peeled and sliced into 1-inch pieces
- 1 can of organic full fat coconut milk
- 2 cups of filtered water
- ½ a bunch of chopped cilantro

Directions

1. Heat the coconut oil over medium heat in a large saucepan.

2. Add the lime zest, garlic, and ginger and cook until they start to turn brown in color, this should take approximately 4 minutes.

3. Add the curry and cook for another 1 minute.

4. Add the coconut milk, water, and sweet potatoes, bring the ingredients to a boil, turn the heat down to low, cover and cook for another 25 minutes.

5. Remove the saucepan from the stove and leave the soup to marinate and cool down for 30 minutes.

6. Pour the soup into a food processor and puree until smooth.

7. Divide into bowls, garnish with lime juice and cilantro and serve.

19: Cauliflower Mashed Potatoes

(Preparation time:30 minutes/Serves: 4 servings)

Ingredients

- 2 teaspoons of coconut oil
- 3 cloves of minced garlic
- 1 chopped onion
- 1 chopped cauliflower head
- 1 chopped carrot
- ¼ cup of yeast-free vegetable broth
- 1 teaspoon of garlic powder
- 2 teaspoons of chopped rosemary
- 2 teaspoons of chopped parsley
- Celtic Grey sea salt
- Black pepper

Directions

1. In a large saucepan heat the coconut oil over medium heat.
2. Add the garlic and onions and sauté until they start to turn brown in color.
3. Add the carrot, cauliflower and vegetable broth. Bring the ingredients to a boil.
4. Turn the heat to low and simmer for 10 minutes.
5. Add the parsley, rosemary, garlic powder, and salt and pepper and cook for a further 5 minutes.
6. Pour the ingredients into a food processor and blend until smooth.
7. Scoop out onto plates and enjoy.

20: Greens Sautéed in Garlic

(Preparation time: 30 minutes /Serves: 2 servings)

Ingredients

- 1 tablespoon of coconut oil
- 3 cloves of finely chopped garlic
- The zest and juice of one lemon
- 1 bunch of leafy greens such as collard greens, spinach or kale
- ½ a cup of yeast-free vegetable broth
- 1 handful of chopped parsley
- Celtic Grey sea salt
- Black pepper

Directions

1. Heat the coconut oil in a large frying pan.
2. Sauté the lemon zest and the garlic for approximately 2 minutes.
3. Add the greens and sauté for a further 2 minutes.
4. Add the vegetable broth, cover and allow the ingredients to steam for a further 5 minutes.
5. Season with salt and black pepper.
6. Drizzle the lemon over the top.
7. Divide onto plates, garnish with parsley and serve.

Dinner Recipes

1: Sesame Asian Noodles With Dressing

(Preparation time: 30 minutes /Serves: 2 servings)

Ingredients for the dressing

- 2 tablespoons of tahini
- 2 teaspoons of gluten-free tamari
- ½ a teaspoon of coconut liquid nectar
- ½ a teaspoon of freshly squeezed lemon juice
- 1 clove of minced garlic

Ingredients for noodles

- 1 chopped scallion
- 1 tablespoon of raw sesame seeds
- 1 thinly sliced carrot
- 1 bag of kelp noodles

Directions

1. Soak the kelp noodles in warm water for 10 minutes until they soften and start to separate.
2. In a mixing bowl, combine the ingredients for the dressing and whisk together thoroughly.
3. Combine the ingredients for the noodles in a large bowl and toss to combine.
4. Pour the dressing over the top of the noodles and toss to combine.

5. Divide onto plates and serve.

2: Sprouted Flavorful Stir Fry

(Preparation time: 30 minutes/Serves: 4 servings)

Ingredients

- 1 ½ cups of quinoa
- 1 clove of minced garlic
- 3 cups of yeast-free vegetable stock

Ingredients for the teriyaki sauce

- ½ a cup of gluten-free tamari
- 1 clove of minced garlic
- 1 teaspoon of minced fresh ginger

Ingredients for the stir fry

- 2 tablespoons of coconut oil
- 2 minced cloves of garlic
- 2 teaspoons of minced fresh ginger
- 1 small white onion
- 1 bunch of broccolini chopped into bite-sized pieces
- 1 stalk of celery cut into chunks
- 8 Brussels sprouts cut into halves
- ½ a bunch of kale chopped into ribbons
- 1 handful of mug bean sprouts

Directions for the quinoa

1. Add the vegetable broth, garlic, and quinoa into a large saucepan, stir to combine and cook on high heat.

2. When the broth begins to boil, turn the heat down to low and allow the ingredients to simmer for 20 minutes. Remove from the cooker and set it to one side.

Directions for the Teriyaki sauce

1. In a small saucepan, combine the ingredients for the teriyaki sauce and simmer until the sauce has reduced by half and it becomes syrupy and thick. Remove from the cooker and set it to one side.

Directions for the stir fry

1. In a large wok or frying pan heat the coconut oil and add the onions, ginger, and garlic. Allow the ingredients to simmer until it turns brown.

2. Add all vegetables apart from the spouts, stir and cover to steam the vegetables for 10 minutes.

3. Divide the quinoa onto plates, and top with stir fry, teriyaki sauce, sprouts and serve.

3: Fennel Soup

(Preparation time: 30 minutes/Serves: 3 servings)

Ingredients

- 2 cups of chopped fennel bulb
- 1 cup of chopped tomato
- 1 ½ tablespoon of fresh lemon juice
- ½ a tablespoon of minced garlic

- ½ a teaspoon of fresh oregano
- ½ a teaspoon of fresh sage
- ½ a teaspoon of Celtic Grey sea salt
- ½ a cup of diced Haas avocado
- ½ a cup of diced cucumber
- 1 cup of diced red pepper
- Extra virgin olive oil

Directions

1. In a food processor combine the sage, oregano, garlic, lemon juice, tomato, fennel, and salt. Blend until smooth.

2. Pour into soup bowls and add the red bell peppers, cucumber, and avocado.

3. Garnish with fresh herbs and olive oil and serve.

4: Asparagus and Adzuki Bean Salad

(Preparation time: 15 minutes/Serves: 2 servings)

Ingredients

- 1 bunch of asparagus with the ends trimmed
- ¼ cup of extra virgin olive oil
- The zest and juice from 1 lemon
- ½ a bunch of chopped parsley
- 1 can of Adzuki beans rinsed and drained
- Celtic Grey sea salt

- Black pepper

Directions

1. Boil a saucepan of water and blanch the asparagus for 8 minutes.

2. Remove the asparagus from the water and use paper towels to pat dry.

3. Chop the asparagus into 1-inch pieces.

4. In a small bowl combine the lemon, olive oil and parsley and whisk together thoroughly.

5. In a large bowl combine the arugula, asparagus, and beans, toss to combine, season with salt and pepper and serve.

5: *Ratatouille*

(Preparation time: 30 minutes/Serves: 4 servings)

Ingredients

- 1 cup of filtered water
- 5 chopped tomatoes
- 1 large zucchini chopped into thin slices
- 1 large eggplant chopped into thin slices
- 1 large chopped onion
- 1 large chopped red bell pepper
- 2 cloves of garlic
- 2 teaspoons of thyme

- 3 tablespoons of coconut oil
- Celtic Grey sea salt
- Black pepper
- 1 cup of steamed quinoa

Directions

1. Heat the coconut oil in a large frying pan over medium heat.

2. Saute the garlic and onions for a few minutes.

3. Add the red bell pepper, zucchini slices, and eggplant and fry for 8 minutes.

4. Add the herbs, tomatoes, and water and, stir to combine and cook for a further 5 minutes.

5. Season with salt and pepper.

6. Divide the quinoa onto plates and top with the ratatouille.

6: Risotto

(Preparation time: 30 minutes/Serves: 4 servings)

Ingredients

- 2 cups of vegetable broth
- 1 cup of quinoa
- 2 tablespoons of coconut oil
- 1 thinly sliced shallot
- 3 cloves of minced garlic

- 1 bunch of Swiss Chard sliced into ribbons
- 1 jar of drained artichoke hearts
- 2 tablespoons of capers
- 1 can of chickpeas
- 1 handful of chopped parsley
- Celtic Grey sea salt
- Black pepper

Directions

1. In a large saucepan, combine the quinoa and the vegetable broth and cook over high heat.

2. Once the broth starts to boil, reduce the temperature to low and simmer for 30 minutes until the liquid has been absorbed.

3. Heat the coconut oil in a large saucepan and cook the shallots for 8 minutes.

4. Add the Swiss Chard and the garlic and cook for 5 minutes.

5. Add the capers, artichokes, and chickpeas and cook for a further 2 minutes.

6. Combine the quinoa and the Swiss chard, season with salt and pepper, stir to combine and divide onto plates and serve.

7: Quinoa and Courgette Salad

(Preparation time: 30 minutes/Serves: 4 servings)

Ingredients

- 1 packet of courgettes washed and sliced
- ½ a cup of quinoa
- 2 tablespoons of olive oil
- 1 teaspoon of cumin
- 1 tin of chickpeas rinsed and drained
- 1 crushed clove of garlic
- 3 tablespoons of extra virgin olive oil
- 2 tablespoons of fresh lemon juice
- 2 finely chopped spring onions
- 1 small handful of chopped flat-leaf parsley

Directions

1. Cook the quinoa in a pot of boiling water over medium heat for 20 minutes until the water has been absorbed. Once cooked remove from the stove and set to one side.

2. In a large saucepan over medium temperature heat the olive oil.

3. Add the courgettes and cook until they become tender and bright green.

4. Remove the courgettes from the saucepan, season and set them to one side.

5. Add the cumin to the saucepan and cook until the fragrance is released, pour this spiced oil on top of the courgettes.

6. In a large bowl combine the parsley, spring onions, lemon juice, extra virgin olive oil, garlic, quinoa, and chickpeas, toss to combine and serve.

8: Gnocchi Cauliflower

(Preparation time: 35 minutes/Serves: 4 servings)

Ingredients for the cauliflower

- 1 cauliflower head cut into florets and steamed
- 1 clove of finely chopped garlic
- 1 cup of flour
- 1 tablespoon of olive oil

Ingredients for the ragout

- 1 tin of whole tomatoes
- 5 thickly sliced courgettes
- ½ a finely sliced onion
- 1 tablespoon of olive oil
- 2 cloves of finely sliced garlic
- 6 large thickly sliced black mushrooms
- 3 cups of vegetable stock
- 1 teaspoon of stevia
- Celtic Grey sea salt
- Black pepper
- Fresh basil for garnish

Directions

1. Blend the garlic and the cauliflower in a food processor until smooth.

2. Add the flour ¼ of a cup at a time, add the salt and continue to blend until the ingredients turn into a soft dough.

3. Sprinkle some flour over a chopping board and transfer the mixture out onto the board and knead the dough until it becomes soft.

4. Slice the dough into four pieces, cover three with a damp cloth and use 1.

5. Roll out the dough into a 3cm rope and cut it into 3cm pieces. Press the pieces down with a fork and set them to one side. Repeat with the other 3 pieces of dough.

6. Heat the olive oil in a frying pan over medium heat and fry the gnocchi on both sides until they are light brown in color.

7. To cook the ragout, heat the olive oil in a large saucepan over medium heat.

8. Add the courgettes, mushrooms, garlic, and onion and fry until golden brown in color.

9. Add the vegetable stock, stevia, and tomatoes. Reduce the heat to low and simmer for 15 minutes.

10. Serve with the cauliflower gnocchi and garnish with basil leaves.

9: Avo Warm Quinoa Salad

(Preparation time: 15 minutes/Serves: 4 servings)

Ingredients

- 4 ripe avocados, peeled and sliced into quarters
- 1 cup of quinoa
- 1 tin of chickpeas rinsed and drained
- 30 grams of torn flat-leaf parsley

Directions

1. Cook the quinoa in boiling water over medium heat for 20 minutes until the water has been absorbed.
2. Add the remaining ingredients into the quinoa and stir to combine.
3. Arrange onto plates and serve.

10: Broccoli and Coconut Thai Soup

(Preparation time: 30 minutes/Serves: 4 servings)

Ingredients

- 50 grams of green curry paste
- 1 can of coconut milk
- 500 ml of water
- 450 grams of chopped broccoli
- 200 grams of baby spinach
- Celtic Grey sea salt
- Black pepper

- 1 diced spring onion
- Coriander leaves

Directions

1. Cook the curry paste in a saucepan over medium heat.

2. Add the water and the coconut oil and bring the ingredients to a boil.

3. Add the broccoli and cook for 10 minutes.

4. Add the spinach and cook for a further 2 minutes.

5. Take the saucepan off the cooker and let the soup cool down.

6. Pour the soup into a food processor and blend until smooth.

7. Add salt and pepper for seasoning.

8. Divide between bowls, garnish with coriander, spinach and spring onions and serve.

11: Swiss Chard and Kale Frittata

(Preparation time: 1 hour/Serves: 4 servings)

Ingredients

- 2 tablespoon of extra virgin olive oil
- 1 finely chopped shallot
- 2 diced leeks
- 1 bunch of rainbow-colored Swiss Chard

- 1 bunch of kale
- The zest of half a lemon
- ½ a teaspoon of ground cumin
- ½ a teaspoon of coriander
- 1 pinch of chili flakes
- 6 eggs
- 100 grams of grated mozzarella
- 60 grams of feta cheese
- Celtic Grey sea salt
- Toasted pine nuts

Directions

1. Preheat the oven to 180 degrees C.

2. Wash the kale and the chard under cold water and pat dry with paper towels.

3. Remove the stems from the chard and the kale and chop the leaves.

4. In a large frying pan heat the oil and then sauté the shallots until lightly browned.

5. Add the leeks and continue to cook for another 2 minutes.

6. Add the kale and the chard and cook until the vegetables begin to wilt.

7. Add the chili, coriander, cumin, and lemon zest and season with salt and pepper.

8. Whisk the eggs in a large bowl and season with salt and pepper.

9. Add the feta cheese, cooked vegetables, and mozzarella and stir to combine.

10. Pour the mixture into a frying pan, sprinkle some pine nuts over the top, cover with foil and bake for 15 minutes. Remove the foil and bake for another 15 minutes.

11. Divide onto plates and serve.

12: Grilled Courgette Salad

(Preparation time: 25 minutes/Serves: 6 servings)

Ingredients

- 6 courgettes thinly sliced
- 80 grams of watercress
- Celtic Grey sea salt

Ingredients for the chili mint dressing

- The juice and zest of ½ a lemon
- 1 red chili, finely chopped, seeds removed
- 15 grams of fresh mint leaves, shredded
- 6 tablespoons of extra virgin olive oil
- Celtic Grey sea salt
- Black pepper

Directions

1. Sprinkle salt over the courgettes to soften them.

2. In a large bowl combine the ingredients for the dressing and whisk together thoroughly.

3. Arrange the watercress on plates, layer with the courgettes and drizzle the dressing over the top.

13: Coconut Milk and Roasted Vegetable Soup

(Preparation time: 50 minutes/Serves: 2 servings)

Ingredients
- 1 chopped cabbage
- 1 chopped butternut
- 1 chopped marrow
- 1 chopped onion
- Chopped green beans
- Olive oil
- Celtic Grey sea salt
- 1 tablespoon of butter
- 1 teaspoon of crushed garlic
- 1 tablespoon of grated ginger
- 1 can of coconut milk
- Black pepper

Directions
1. Preheat the oven to 180 degrees C.

2. Spread the chopped vegetables out into a baking tray.

3.   Drizzle olive oil over the top and season with salt and pepper

4.   Roast for 40 minutes.

5.   Heat the butter over medium heat and sauté the ginger and garlic.

6.   Add the coconut milk and boil on medium temperature for 30 minutes.

7.   Pour the coconut milk into a bowl, add the roasted vegetables and season with salt and pepper.

8.   Divide into bowls and serve.

14: Quinoa Crunchy Salad

(Preparation time: 50 minutes/Serves: 4 servings)

Ingredients

- 2 cups of quinoa
- 1 butternut squash
- 1 head of cauliflower
- Olive oil
- 2 cucumbers sliced into wedges
- 2 sliced carrots
- 1 bunch of chopped kale
- 1 bunch of chopped mint
- 1 block of feta cheese, crumbled
- ½ a cup of roasted pumpkin seeds

- ½ a cup of lentil sprouts
- Celtic Grey sea salt
- Black pepper

Ingredients for the vinaigrette

- Olive oil
- ½ a cup of white wine vinegar
- The molasses from 1 pomegranate
- ¼ cup of wholegrain mustard
- The juice of 1 lemon
- ½ a cup of parsley
- Celtic Grey sea salt
- Black pepper

Directions

1. Heat the olive oil in a frying pan and fry the cauliflower until browned.

2. Transfer all of the ingredients for the vinaigrette into a food processor and blend until smooth.

3. In a large bowl combine the ingredients for the salad and toss together.

4. Divide the salad into bowls and drizzle with the vinaigrette and serve.

15: Pesto Kale Pasta

(Preparation time: 20 minutes/Serves: 4 servings)

Ingredients

- 1 bunch of kale
- 2 cups of fresh basil
- ¼ cup of extra virgin olive oil
- ½ a cup of walnuts soaked overnight
- 2 freshly squeezed limes
- Celtic Grey sea salt
- Black pepper
- 2 zucchinis
- Sliced asparagus
- 1 cup of cherry tomatoes halved

Directions

1. Put all of the ingredients except the zucchinis into a food processor and blend until smooth.
2. Spiralize the zucchinis to make noodles.
3. Divide the zucchini noodles onto plates and top with the pesto, asparagus and cherry tomatoes.

16: *Burrito Quinoa Bowl*

(Preparation time: 30 minutes/Serves: 4 servings)

Ingredients

- 1 cup of quinoa
- 2 cans of black beans
- 4 sliced green onions

- The juice from 2 limes
- 4 cloves of minced garlic
- 1 teaspoon of cumin
- 2 sliced avocados
- 1 handful of chopped cilantro

Directions

1. Cook the quinoa for 20 minutes in boiling water over medium heat. While it is boiling add the cumin, garlic, lime juice, and onions. Simmer until all the water has been absorbed.
2. Divide the quinoa onto dishes and top with cilantro, avocado, and beans.

17: Quinoa Thai Salad

(Preparation time: 30 minutes/Serves: 4 servings)

Ingredients for the dressing

1. 1 tablespoon of sesame seeds
2. 1 teaspoon of chopped garlic
3. 1 teaspoon of freshly squeezed lemon juice
4. 3 teaspoons of apple cider vinegar
5. 2 teaspoons of gluten-free tamari
6. ¼ cup of tahini
7. 1 pitted date
8. 1 teaspoon of Celtic Grey sea salt

9.   ½ a teaspoon of toasted sesame oil

Ingredients for the salad

- 1 cup of steamed quinoa
- Arugula, 1 large handful
- 1 sliced tomato
- ¼ diced red onion

Directions

1.   To make the dressing combine all the ingredients into a food processor and blend until smooth.

2.   Steam the quinoa in boiling water for 20 minutes and set it to one side.

3.   In a large bowl, combine the quinoa red onions, sliced tomatoes, and arugula and toss to combine.

4.   Divide onto plates, drizzle the dressing over the top and serve.

18: Sesame Asian Noodles

(Preparation time: 30 minutes/Serves: 4 servings)

Ingredients for the dressing

- 2 tablespoons of tahini
- 2 teaspoons of gluten-free tamari
- ½ a teaspoon of liquid coconut nectar
- ½ a teaspoon of freshly squeezed lemon juice
- 1 clove of minced garlic

Ingredients for the noodle salad

- 1 chopped scallion
- 1 tablespoon of raw sesame seeds
- 1 chopped red bell pepper
- 1 bag of kelp noodles

Directions

1. Combine the ingredients for the dressing in a small bowl and whisk together thoroughly.

2. Soak the kelp noodles in boiling water for 10 minutes and then drain the water.

3. Add the scallions, sesame seeds, and red bell pepper to the noodles and toss to combine.

4. Divide the noodles onto plates, drizzle with the dressing and serve.

19: Alfredo Pasta

(Preparation time: 30 minutes/Serves: 4 servings)

Ingredients For The Alfredo Cauliflower Sauce

- 1 large cauliflower head, roughly chopped
- 1 finely sliced yellow onion
- 1 finely chopped clove of garlic
- 2 tablespoons of extra virgin olive oil
- Celtic Grey sea salt
- 1 can of white beans, drained and rinsed

- 1/3 cup of yeast-free vegetable broth
- 1 cup of almond milk
- 1 teaspoon of freshly squeezed lemon juice
- ¼ teaspoon of smoked paprika
- Black pepper

Ingredients For The Noodles

- 2-4 zucchinis depending on how much you want to make
- ½ a tablespoon of coconut oil
- ¼ cup of filtered water
- 8 cups of baby spinach
- 12 thinly sliced sun-dried tomatoes

Directions

- To make the alfredo cauliflower sauce start by preheating the oven to 400 degrees F.
- Combine the garlic, yellow onion and cauliflower in a large bowl, drizzle the extra virgin olive oil over the top, sprinkle with sea salt and toss to combine.
- Arrange the vegetables in a single layer onto a baking tray and roast for 45 to 60 minutes.
- Once the vegetables are cooked, remove them from the oven and pour them into a food processor. Add the vegetable broth, white beans, almond milk, smoked paprika, lemon juice, and black pepper and blend until the ingredients become creamy and smooth.

- If you need to adjust the consistency add more broth or milk, season with salt and pepper and set to one side.

20: Dinner: Winter Veggie Soup

(Preparation time: 30 minutes/Serves: 4 servings)

Ingredients

- 3 tablespoons of coconut oil
- 3 leeks, remove the green part and slice them thinly
- 2 carrots
- 1 thinly sliced fennel bulb
- 4 cloves of minced garlic
- 2 fresh sprigs of finely chopped rosemary
- 1 cup of savoy cabbage thinly sliced
- 6 cups of vegetable stock
- 1 can of rinsed beans rinsed and drained
- 1 handful of chopped flat-leaf parsley
- Celtic Grey sea salt

Directions

1. Heat the oil in a large saucepan over low to medium heat.
2. Add the fennel, carrots, and leeks and cook for approximately 8 minutes until the leeks become slightly brown in color and soft.

3. Add the rosemary and garlic and cook for another minute.

4. Add the garlic and continue to cook for a further 1 minute.

5. Add the beans and the stock and bring the ingredients to a boil for 15 minutes.

6. Season with salt and pepper, add the parsley and serve.

21: Dinner: Coconut Curry

(Preparation time: 30 minutes/Serves: 4 servings)

Ingredients for the quinoa

- 1 cup of quinoa
- 2 cups of yeast-free vegetable broth
- Celtic Grey sea salt

Ingredients for the coconut curry

- 4 cups of zucchini sliced into cubes
- 1 cup of green peas
- 2 cups of coconut milk
- 1 chopped onion
- 2 cloves of minced garlic
- ½ a cup of filtered water
- 2 tablespoons of curry powder
- ½ a teaspoon of Celtic Grey sea salt

Directions

1. To cook the quinoa add 2 cups of vegetable broth and 1 cup of quinoa into a saucepan, season with salt and bring to a boil over medium heat. Turn the temperature down to low and cook for 15 minutes until the quinoa has absorbed the vegetable broth.

2. Pour the coconut milk into a medium-sized saucepan and heat over high heat.

3. Add the garlic and the onions and cook for 5 minutes.

4. Add the curry powder and cook for another 2 minutes.

5. Add the water and the zucchini and simmer for a further 15 minutes.

6. Add the peas, season with salt and cook for another 1 minute.

7. Arrange the quinoa onto plates and pour, pour the coconut curry over the top and serve.

Dessert recipes

1: Tropical Frozen Chocolate Monkey

(Preparation time: 30 minutes /Serves: 2 servings)

Ingredients

- 2 frozen bananas
- 2 tablespoons of coconut oil
- 2 tablespoons of cacao powder
- 1 tablespoon of cacao nibs
- 2 tablespoons of chia seeds
- 2 cups of coconut milk

Directions

1. Blend all the ingredients until smooth except the chia seeds in a food processor.
2. Add the chia seeds and pulse a few times.
3. Transfer into bowls and serve.

2: Summer Fruit Mixed Salad

(Preparation time: 30 minutes/Serves: 4 servings)

(Preparation time: /Serves: 4 servings)

Ingredients

- 1 chopped pitted peach
- 1 chopped pitted nectarine

- ½ a cup of cherries, seeds and stems removed
- ½ a cup of blueberries
- The juice and zest of one lemon
- 1 teaspoon of chopped mint
- 1 heaping tablespoon of coconut butter

Directions

1. Combine all the ingredients in a large bowl and toss to combine.
2. Divide into bowls and serve.

3: Alkaline Macaroons

(Preparation time: 30 minutes /Serves: 20 macaroons)

Ingredients

- 1 cup of raw almonds
- 1 cup of coconut flakes, unsweetened
- 1 cup of apricots
- 3 teaspoons of cardamom
- ½ a teaspoon of vanilla extract

Directions

1. Transfer all ingredients into a food processor and blend for 2 minutes until smooth.
2. Use your hands to mold the batter into macaroons.
3. Arrange the macaroons onto dehydrator sheets

4. Set the dehydrator to 115 degrees F and dehydrate for 3-4 hours.

5. Serve with coconut butter or almond butter.

6. If you don't have a dehydrator you can heat them in a toaster oven or you can eat them raw.

4: Sweet Sesame Treat

(Preparation time: 30 minutes /Serves: 15-20 balls)

Ingredients

- ½ a cup of raw almonds
- ½ a cup of sesame seeds
- 6 dates
- 3 tablespoons of tahini
- 1 teaspoon of coconut oil
- ½ a teaspoon of Celtic Grey sea salt
- ½ a teaspoon of vanilla extract
- 1 tablespoon of coconut sugar
- 4 teaspoons of stevia
- Cacao powder

Directions

1. Transfer all the ingredients apart from the sesame seeds into a food processor and blend for a few minutes until oil is released.

2. Pour the blended ingredients out into a mixing bowl.

3. Add 2 tablespoons of sesame seeds and stir to combine.

4. Form the mixture into balls by molding them with your hands.

5. Pour some sesame seeds onto a plate and roll the balls in them.

6. Dust them in cacao powder and then leave them in the fridge to harden.

5: Chocolate Avocado Mousse

(Preparation time: 1 hour 10 minutes Serves: 2 servings)

Ingredients

- 1 ½ chopped Haas avocado
- 2/3 cup of coconut water
- 1 tablespoon of vanilla
- 2 tablespoons of raw cacao
- 3 dates
- 1 ½ teaspoon of Celtic sea salt

Directions

1. Transfer all ingredients into a food processor and blend until smooth.

2. Transfer the blended mixture into a bowl and leave in the fridge for 1 hour.

6: Coconut Vanilla Chia Pudding

(Preparation time: 5 hours 10 minutes/Serves: 4 servings)

Ingredients

- 2 cups of coconut water
- ½ a cup of cashews
- 2 tablespoons of coconut oil
- 1 teaspoon of cinnamon
- 3 medium dates
- 1/8 teaspoon of Celtic Grey sea salt
- 2 teaspoons of vanilla
- 6 tablespoons of chia seeds

Directions

1. Blend all ingredients except the chia seeds in a food processor.

2. Add the chia seeds and blend at a low speed.

3. Pour the pudding into an airtight container and place in the fridge for 5 hours.

4. Garnish with cinnamon before serving.

7: Banana and Chocolate Fro Yo

(Preparation time:20 minutes/Serves:2 servings)

Ingredients

- 2 frozen bananas

- 3 tablespoons of raw cacao powder
- 1 tablespoon of raw almond butter
- ¼ cup of unsweetened almond milk
- 1 tablespoon of hemp seeds

Directions
- Blend the banana and cacao in a food processor.
- Slowly add the almond milk and continue to blend.
- Pour the mixture into bowls, sprinkle with hemp seeds and serve.

8: Chopped Berries With Coconut Butter and Mint

(Preparation time: 15 minutes/Serves: 1 serving)

Ingredients
- 1 cup of mixed berries (raspberries, strawberries, and blueberries)
- 2 tablespoons of melted coconut butter
- 1 tablespoon of chopped mint

Directions
1. Put the berries into a small bowl.
2. Drizzle the coconut butter over the top, garnish with mint and eat.

9: Cinnamon Ginger Fruit With Tahini Sweet Dip

(Preparation time: 10 minutes/Serves: 2 servings)

Ingredients

- 1 chopped pear
- 1 chopped apple
- 3 tablespoons of grated ginger
- 1 teaspoon of cinnamon
- 1 teaspoon of Celtic Grey sea salt

Ingredients for the Tahini sweet dip

- 3 tablespoons of tahini
- 3 tablespoons of raw almond butter
- 1 tablespoon of coconut liquid nectar
- 2 tablespoons of coconut oil
- 2 teaspoons of wheat-free tamari
- ¼ teaspoon of cayenne

Directions

1. Combine all of the ingredients for the tahini dip into a food processor and blend until smooth.

2. Put the pear, apple, and ginger into a bowl and toss to combine.

3. Pour the dip over the top and serve.

10: Berry Quinoa Cobbler

(Preparation time: 30 minutes/Serves: 4 servings)

Ingredients

- ½ a cup of cooked quinoa
- 1 cup of rolled oats, gluten-free
- ½ a cup of quinoa flour
- ½ a cup of chopped cashews
- ½ a cup of coconut oil
- ¼ cup of ground flax seeds
- 1 teaspoon of vanilla
- ¼ cup of coconut milk
- 1 teaspoon of cinnamon
- 4 chopped dates
- 3 cups of mixed berries
- Coconut butter

Directions

1. Preheat the oven to 375 degrees C.
2. Cook the quinoa in a saucepan of boiling water for 20 minutes until all the water has been absorbed.
3. Combine all the ingredients (including the quinoa) apart from the berries into a large mixing bowl.
4. Pour the berries into a baking dish and cover with the oats quinoa mixture. Bake for 40 minutes until the top becomes golden brown in color.
5. Serve with a spoonful of coconut butter.

11: Super Soy Pudding

(Preparation time: 10 minutes/Serves: 2 servings)

Ingredients

- 1 cup of unsweetened almond milk
- 2 diced avocados
- 2 scoops of super soy powder
- Stevia
- 8 ice cubes

Directions

1. Transfer all of the ingredients into a food processor and blend until smooth.
2. Pour out into bowls and serve.

12: Buckwheat Sprouted Flatties

(Preparation time: 8 hours 10 minutes/Serves: 12 servings)

Ingredients

- 3 cups of sprouted buckwheat soaked overnight
- 1/3 cup of essential balance oil
- 2 teaspoons of garlic herb bread seasonings
- 1-2 teaspoons of Celtic Grey sea salt
- 1 teaspoon of All-Purpose Chefs Shake

Directions

1. Transfer all of the ingredients into a food processor and blend until smooth.

2. Pour the mixture into a plastic-lined dehydrator tray. Spread the batter out with a spatula so that it's half an inch thick.

3. Place in the dehydrator for 8 hours on 100 degrees C.

4. Remove from the tray from the dehydrator and transfer the flattie onto a mesh-lined tray and continue to dehydrate for a further 1 hour until they are completely crisp and dry.

5. Slice into squares and store in an airtight container.

13: Granola

(Preparation time: 37 hours/Serves: 12 servings)

Ingredients

- 2 cups of almonds soaked overnight in filtered water
- 1 cup of pecans soaked in filtered water for 1 hour
- 1 cup of walnuts soaked in filtered water for 1 hour
- 1 cup of macadamia nuts
- 1 cup of pine nuts
- 2 cups of dried coconut
- 1 ¼ cups of Mesquite flour
- 1 1/3 cup of ground cinnamon

- ½ a tablespoon of Celtic Grey sea salt
- 3 tablespoons of stevia
- Honey for topping

Directions

1. Combine the coconut flakes, almonds, pecans and walnuts in a food processor and blend.

2. Pour it out into a large bowl and set to one side.

3. Combine the remaining ingredients into the same bowl and toss to combine.

4. Pour out onto a dehydrator sheet and dehydrate for 36 hours at 110 degrees.

5. Cut into squares and store serve with honey or a topping of your choice.

14: Nutty Almond Pie Crust

(Preparation time: 30 minutes/Serves: 4 servings)

Ingredients for the pie crust

- ½ a cup of spelled flakes ground into a flour
- ¼ cup of ground flax meal
- 1 tablespoon of arrowroot powder
- ½ a teaspoon of ground cinnamon
- 1/8 teaspoon of ground cloves
- 1 packet of stevia powder
- 1 teaspoon of vanilla

- 2 tablespoons of coconut butter
- 2 tablespoons of water

Ingredients for the filling

- 2 cups of mixed berries.
- 1 tablespoon of stevia
- ¼ cup of honey
- Coconut butter

Directions

1. In a large bowl combine all of the dry ingredients.

2. In another large bowl combine all of the wet ingredients and whisk to combine.

3. Pour the wet ingredients over the dry ingredients and whisk to combine.

4. Scoop the mixture out into a pie plate and use your fingers to press it around the sides and along the bottom.

5. Place the pie plate into the oven and bake for 20 minutes.

6. In a large bowl combine the berries, stevia, and honey and stir to combine.

7. Remove from the oven and fill with the berry mixture, put back in the oven and bake for 10 minutes.

8. Top with coconut butter and serve.

15: Creamy Pumpkin Pie

(Preparation time: 1 hour/Serves: 6-8 servings)

Ingredients for the filling

- 12 ounces of tofu
- 2 cups of fresh pumpkin
- 2 teaspoons of vanilla
- 2 teaspoons of cinnamon
- ¼ teaspoon of Celtic Grey sea salt
- ¾ teaspoons of nutmeg
- ¼ teaspoon of cloves
- ½ teaspoon of ginger
- ¼ teaspoon of stevia
- 3 tablespoons of psyllium

Ingredients for the pie crust

- ½ a cup of spelled flakes ground into a flour
- ¼ cup of ground flax meal
- 1 tablespoon of arrowroot powder
- ½ a teaspoon of ground cinnamon
- 1/8 teaspoon of ground cloves
- 1 packet of stevia powder
- 1 teaspoon of vanilla
- 2 tablespoons of coconut butter
- 2 tablespoons of water

Directions for the pie crust

1. In a large bowl combine all of the dry ingredients.

2.   In another large bowl combine all of the wet ingredients and whisk to combine.

3.   Pour the wet ingredients over the dry ingredients and whisk to combine.

4.   Scoop the mixture out into a pie plate and use your fingers to press it around the sides and along the bottom.

5.   Place the pie plate into the oven and bake for 20 minutes.

Directions for the filling

1.   Combine the stevia, ginger, cloves, nutmeg, salt, cinnamon, vanilla, pumpkin and tofu in a food processor. Blend until creamy and smooth.

2.   Add the psyllium and continue to blend.

3.   Scoop into the almond crust pie and put it into the fridge for an hour.

4.   Top with whipped tofu whipped cream and serve.

16: Oatmeal Quinoa Rasin Cookies

(Preparation time: 23 minutes/Serves: 9 servings)

Ingredients

- ½ a cup of cooked quinoa
- 2/3 cups of rolled oats
- 2 tablespoons of oat flour
- 2/3 cup of raisins
- ¼ cup of raisins

- 1/3 cup of water
- 1 teaspoon of cinnamon

Directions

1. Preheat the oven to 350 degrees F.

2. Combine the water and the 2/3 of raisins into a food processor and blend until smooth.

3. Combine the cinnamon, oat flour, oats, quinoa, and raisin paste in a large bowl and whisk together thoroughly.

4. Lin a baking sheet with parchment paper.

5. Roll the batter into balls and arrange them onto the baking sheet and then flatten them into cookie shapes. Put them into the oven and bake for 14 minutes.

6. Take them out of the oven and leave them to cool down for 10 minutes before serving.

17: Oatmeal Banana Cookies

(Preparation time: 15 minutes/Serves: 10 servings)

Ingredients

- 2 large ripe bananas
- 1 cup of oats
- ½ a cup of raisins

Directions

1. Preheat the oven to 350 degrees C.

2. Break the bananas up and place them into a bowl, use the back of a fork to mash them.

3. Add the raisins and the oats and whisk together thoroughly.

4. Roll the batter into balls.

5. Line a baking tray with parchment paper.

6. Arrange the balls onto the baking tray and flatten into the shape of cookies.

7. Bake for 12 minutes.

8. Remove from the oven and serve.

18: Desert: Strawberry Ice-cream

(Preparation time: 30 minutes/Serves: 4 servings)

Ingredients

- 2 large bananas
- 1 cup of coconut milk
- ½ a cup of fresh strawberries
- 2 cups of ice
- 2 teaspoons of chia seeds
- 2 tablespoons of coconut flakes, unsweetened
- 1 tablespoon of goji berries
- 1 tablespoon of hemp seeds
- 1 scoop of Alkamind Daily Minerals
- Mint leaves for garnish

Directions

1. Blend the ice, Alkamind Daily Minerals, chia seeds, strawberries, coconut milk and banana in a food processor until smooth.

2. Add the goji berries and continue to blend until smooth.

3. Pour the ice-cream into a freezer-proof bowl and sprinkle hemp seeds and coconut flakes over the top and leave the container in the freezer for 2 hours.

4. When ready to serve, remove from the freezer, sprinkle with mint leaves and eat.

19: Dessert: Apple Crumble and Spiced Pear

(Preparation time: 30 minutes/Serves: 4 servings)

Ingredients

- 1 tablespoon of coconut oil
- 1 sliced green apple
- 1 sliced pear
- 1 teaspoon of cinnamon
- ½ a teaspoon of nutmeg
- ¼ cup of rolled oats, gluten-free
- ¼ cup of raw, chopped almonds

Directions

- Heat the coconut oil in a large saucepan and add the sliced pears, apples, nutmeg, and cinnamon. Cook for approximately 5 minutes until the fruit becomes tender.

- Divide the fruit into bowls and top with almonds, oats and a dash of cinnamon.

20: Dessert: Chia Pumpkin Pudding

(Preparation time: 30 minutes/Serves: 4 servings)

Ingredients

- 2 cups of coconut water
- ½ a cup of cashews
- ¼ cup of fresh pumpkin puree
- 2 tablespoons of coconut oil
- 1 tablespoon of coconut flakes, unsweetened
- 1 teaspoon of cinnamon
- ¼ teaspoon of nutmeg
- 3 dates, medium-sized
- 1/8 teaspoon of Celtic Gray salt
- 2 teaspoons of vanilla
- 6 tablespoons of chia seeds
- Nutmeg/cinnamon for garnish

Directions

1. Place all of the ingredients into a food processor except the chia seeds and blend until smooth.

2.   Set the food processor on the lowest setting and slowly add the chia seeds.

3.   Pour the mixture into an airtight container and leave it in the fridge for a minimum of 5 hours prior to serving.

4.   Garnish with nutmeg or cinnamon

21: Dessert: Raw Pumpkin Pie

(Preparation time: 30 minutes /Serves: 6 servings)

Ingredients for the pie crust

- 1 cup of raw almonds
- 1 cup of coconut flakes, unsweetened
- 1 cup of dates
- 1 teaspoon of cinnamon

Ingredients for the pie filling

- 1 cup of pecans (soaked overnight)
- 1 ¼ cups of organic pumpkin puree
- 6 dates
- ½ a teaspoon of cinnamon
- ½ a teaspoon of nutmeg
- ¼ teaspoon of Celtic Grey sea salt
- 1 teaspoon of vanilla
- 1 teaspoon of Tamari, gluten-free (optional)

Directions for the pie crust

1. Blend the ingredients for the pie crust in a food processor until the oils are released from the mixture and the ingredients begin to stick together.

2. Scoop the mixture out into a pie pan or a tart mold. First, mold the mixture along the sides and then mold it along the bottom so that it sticks properly

Directions for the filling

1. Add all the ingredients, except the cinnamon into a food processor and blend until smooth.

2. Fill in the pie crust with the mixture.

3. Sprinkle the cinnamon over the top and put the pie in the fridge to mold and chill.

Drink Recipes

1: Mayan Dairy-Free Hot Chocolate

(Preparation time: 5 minutes/ Serves: 2 servings)

Ingredients

- 2 cups of unsweetened almond milk
- ¼ cup of raw cacao
- 1 tablespoon of cinnamon
- A dash of cayenne pepper (optional)

Directions

1. Combine all the ingredients into a food processor and blend until smooth.
2. Transfer the pureed mixture into a saucepan and heat.
3. Pour into glasses and serve.

2: Watermelon Gazpacho

(Preparation time: 30 minutes /Serves: 4 servings)

Ingredients

- 1 watermelon, remove the rind and chop into bite-sized pieces
- ¼ cup of cilantro leaves, plus additional for garnishing
- 3 tablespoons of freshly squeezed lime juice

- 2 tablespoons of mint leaves plus more for garnish
- 1 cucumber
- 2 tablespoons of extra virgin olive oil
- 1 jalapeno, chopped and stemmed
- 1 heirloom tomato, large, chopped and cored
- 1 chopped shallot
- Celtic Grey sea salt
- Black pepper

Directions

1. Transfer the shallot, tomato, jalapeno, cucumber, olive oil, mint, lime juice, cilantro and watermelon to a food processor. Blend until smooth, transfer into a large bowl and refrigerate for at least 4 hours.

2. When ready to serve divide into bowls and garnish with fresh cilantro and mint leaves.

3: Green pH Booster Juice

(Preparation time: 10 minutes/Serves: 2 servings)

Ingredients

- 2 chopped cucumbers
- 4 chopped celery stalks
- ½ a peeled lemon

Directions

1. Add all of the ingredients to a juicer and blend.

2.   Pour out into glasses and drink.

4: Alkaline Lemonade

(Preparation time: 30 minutes /Serves: 4 servings)

Ingredients

- 3 peeled lemons, seeds removed
- 3 tablespoons of coconut oil
- 1 green apple, cored
- 6 cups of filtered water
- 1 teaspoon of Celtic Grey sea salt
- A few drops of organic liquid stevia
- 1 teaspoon of grated ginger (optional)
- A pinch of cayenne pepper (optional)

Directions

1.   Transfer all ingredients into a food processor and blend until juiced.

2.   Pour the lemonade into glasses and serve.

5: Cashew Chocolate Milk

(Preparation time: 15 minutes/Serves: 2 servings)

Ingredients

- 1 cup of cashews
- 1 cup of water

- 3 cups of water
- 1 teaspoon of vanilla
- 1 teaspoon of cinnamon
- ½ a teaspoon of sea salt
- ¼ cup of cacao powder
- 1 tablespoon of coconut oil
- 1 tablespoon of coconut butter
- Cacao nibs for garnish

Directions

1. Blend 1 cup of water and 1 cup of cashews in a food processor.
2. Add the rest of the ingredients and continue to blend until smooth.
3. Pour into glasses, add a handful of ice cubes and garnish with cacao nibs.

6: Hemp Milk

(Preparation time: 10 minutes/Serves: 2 servings)

Ingredients

- 1 cup of shelled hemp seeds
- 2 cups of filtered water
- ½ a teaspoon of vanilla extract
- ½ a tablespoon of coconut oil
- 1/8 teaspoon of Celtic Grey sea salt

- Cheesecloth
- 2 tablespoons of cacao powder
- ½ a teaspoon of cinnamon
- ½ a banana

Directions

1. Put the seeds into a food processor; add some water 1 inch above the seeds. Blend the seeds until they become thick and creamy.

2. Add the remaining ingredients (except the cheesecloth) and blend until smooth.

3. Strain through a cheesecloth into a large bowl.

4. Pour into glasses and serve.

7: Lavender Cucumber Infused Water

(Preparation time: 12 hours 10 minutes/Serves: 2 servings)

Ingredients

- 8 cups of filtered water
- 1 teaspoon of dried lavender
- 1 thinly sliced small cucumber

Directions

1. Transfer all the ingredients into a pitcher and leave it in the fridge for 12 hours so that the ingredients infuse into the water.

8: Mint Watermelon Infused Water

(Preparation time: 12 hours 10 minutes/Serves 2 servings)

Ingredients

- 8 cups of filtered water
- 2 cups of cubed watermelon
- 3 sprigs of mint

Directions

1. Transfer all the ingredients into a pitcher and leave it in the fridge for 12 hours so that the ingredients infuse into the water.

9: Detox Water

(Preparation time: 12 hours 10 minutes/Serves: 10 servings)

Ingredients

- A jug of filtered water
- 1 sliced lemon
- 1 thinly sliced medium cucumber
- A handful of mint leaves
- 1 quarter of a grapefruit

Directions

1. Transfer all the ingredients into a pitcher and leave it in the fridge for 12 hours so that the ingredients infuse into the water.

10: Mojito Water

(Preparation time: 12 hours 10 minutes/Serves: 10 servings)

Ingredients

- A jug of filtered water
- 1 sliced lemon
- 2 slices of lime
- 1 thinly sliced medium cucumber
- A handful of mint leaves

Directions

1. Transfer all the ingredients into a pitcher and leave it in the fridge for 12 hours so that the ingredients infuse into the water.

11: Lemon, Ginger, and Tumeric Tea

(Preparation times: 20 minutes/Serves: 3 servings)

Ingredients

- 16-20 ounces of filtered water
- 1 inch of peeled and diced organic turmeric root
- 1 inch of peeled and diced organic ginger root

- Black pepper
- 1 slice of lemon

Directions

1. Boil a pot of water and then remove it from the cooker.

2. Add the ginger, turmeric and black pepper, stir to combine and leave it to soak for at least 10 minutes. (The longer you leave it the more concentrated and potent the tea will be).

3. Pour the tea into cups, add the lemon slice and serve.

12: Zinger Green Juice

(Preparation time: 10 minutes/Serves: 2 servings)

Ingredients

- 2 cucumbers
- 1 lemon
- A 2-inch piece of ginger
- A handful of string beans
- 2 pears
- 2 tablespoons of chia seeds

Directions

1. Add all of the ingredients into a food processor and blend until smooth.

2. Pour into glasses and serve.

13: Sweet Green Alkaline Juice

(Preparation time: 10 minutes/Serves: 2 servings)

Ingredients

- 1 bunch of Swiss Chard, stems removed)
- A handful of fresh mint
- 1 cucumber
- 1 pear
- 1 tablespoon of chia seeds

Direcions

1. Add all ingredients into a juicer and juice.
2. Pour into glasses and serve.

Conclusion

I want to thank you once again for purchasing my book and even more so for getting to the end of it. I hope that the information you have read has served you well and that not only will you use it for yourself but you will educate others also.

Call me an optimist but I believe that we can beat cancer. However, it is going to take a focused and concentrated effort to educate ourselves on what is causing this detestable disease and taking the necessary steps to prevent and cure it.

I wish you all the best on your journey to total health and healing!

One last thing!

I want to give you a **one-in-two-hundred chance** to win a **$200.00 Amazon Gift card** as a thank-you for reading this book.

All I ask is that you give me some feedback, so I can improve this or my next book :)

ELIZABETH A. COHEN

Your opinion is *super valuable* to me. It will only take a minute of your time to let me know what you like and what you didn't like about this book. The hardest part is deciding how to spend the two hundred dollars! Just follow this link.

http://reviewers.win/alkalinecancer

Made in United States
Troutdale, OR
08/16/2024

22032036R00080